The Ultimate Nutribullet Smoothie Recipe Guide

by Neo Monefa

THANK YOU FOR DOWNLOADING! IF YOU ENJOYED THIS BOOK AND WOULD LIKE TO READ MORE TITLES FROM MY COLLECTION CLICK THIS LINK

Table of Contents

1. **Introduction**

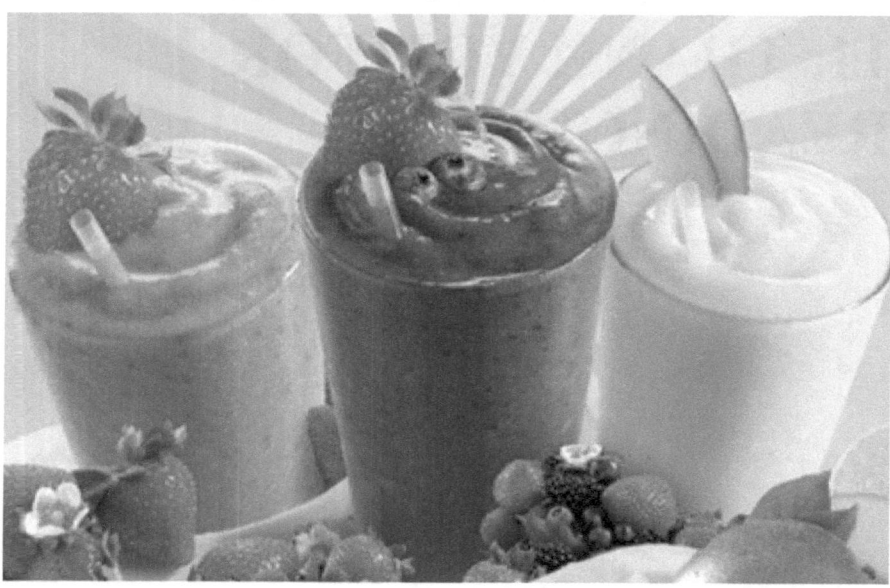

Smoothies are the real deal when it comes to having a diet that not only tastes delightful but also has great nutritive value. Being composed of fruits, natural herbs and all kinds of amazing elements, smoothies are a "must include" item in your daily diet. So, here I am with a wonderful variety of smoothie recipes for you to try!

The best thing about these recipes is that they only require some 'magical mixing' of ingredients and a little blending in your nutribullet and voila! Whether you need a smoothie to lose some extra pounds or you are looking for something to detoxify your body, the solution lies right here. The recipes include a whole bunch of healthy things like cinnamon, apples, oranges, broccoli, lime, blueberries, spinach etc. Everything has its unique advantage; some are known to burn down the 'troubling' layers of fats while others cleanse your body from all kinds of toxic stuff. There is good news for age conscious people as well. Now, you don't have to try any weird methods to slow down the process of aging. Just try out "My Age Prevention Smoothies" and you'll know the difference.

The recipes in this book have been gathered from culinary experts and nutritionists who just love to experiment and create sensational stuff. Also, these smoothies are very easy to make!!

2. Health Benefits of Smoothies

We live in a very fast moving world where we don't even spare time for our families let alone for maintaining our health. Most of the people 'fuel' themselves using junk food like hamburgers, pizzas, burritos, etc. How can they expect to gain all the necessary vitamins and minerals through these things? For such people, smoothies are the most viable option. They can be made instantly and you can have them quickly before doing whatever it is that you do.

Necessary Vitamins and Minerals:

Vitamins and minerals are essential for human body. The most common sources are seasonal fruits and vegetables but people generally do not take these things on daily basis.

Vital elements like vitamin C, folate and potassium can be obtained from citrus fruits like oranges, lemons and from tropical fruits which include papaya, pineapple, avocados, coconut, pomegranates, bananas and mangoes. These fruits are widely used in smoothies because they taste good and they provide you with numerous health benefits. These fruits are the main ingredients of the recipes included in this book.

Vitamin C is known to boost up the immune system by helping in the synthesis of collagen, a protein that forms blood clots, muscular and arterial structures and ligaments. Potassium on the other hand is crucial for healthy functioning of heart muscles and regulating blood pressure. It also prevents the formation of oxalic acid, a nasty compound that causes kidney stones.

Folate is also a very important element that enhances cellular health and repairs the worn out tissues of the body. Some of the above mentioned fruits are also rich in manganese and beta carotene. Magnesium is very important for our skeletal structures, nerves and thyroid glands. Beta carotene is crucial for eyes and it boosts up the natural defense of our body against bacteria and viruses.

Fiber:

For those of you who don't know the importance of fiber; let me tell you that you simply can't digest your food without it. An average person requires about 25 to 38 grams of fiber per day depending upon the age and sex. Well, if you are facing problems like constipation, weight gain, high blood and sugar levels and nausea, then you seriously need to get yourself a load of fiber. And what better way to do so than by having a yummy fruit or green smoothie. Your preference should be to try smoothies that are composed of blackberries, pears, apples, melons, celery, kale or beet leaves.

Water:

"Water is life." This quote is true to its core. Your body would simply cease to function properly due to the lack of water. Drinking fruit or green smoothies is a good way not only to stay hydrated but also to fulfill your nutritional requirements. Your blood flow will remain normal, thus saving you from problems like high blood pressure and formation of clots in the blood vessels. Also, your excretion mechanisms would work effectively and you won't have to face problems like constipation, kidney stones, bladder infections, etc. It is said that staying hydrated slows down aging so you should definitely try these smoothies. Who knows you might actually live longer and healthier.

Antioxidants:

Antioxidants are crucial for one's health. If you want to stay away from cancers, heart problems, DNA degeneration and several common diseases, then your diet must have an adequate quantity of antioxidants. Lucky for you, my smoothie recipes are solely comprised of fruits and vegetables that are rich in antioxidant minerals.

The most common antioxidants are macro-minerals like magnesium, calcium, sodium, potassium, sulfur, phosphorus, etc. Other types of antioxidants are vitamins C and E. All of these minerals and vitamins are abundant in fresh green vegetables like kale, celery, spinach, cucumber and in tropical and citrus fruits like blueberries, raspberries, oranges, strawberries, mangoes, avocados, coconut, etc.

3. About Making Smoothies with the Nutribullet

Say goodbye to your old and slow blender which has given you nothing but a headache every time you process something in it. It's time to buy a Nutribullet and know what it feels like to blend anything in seconds. Nutribullet is a 600 watt, high speed blender that makes your blending experience wonderful. Whether you need to process leafy green vegetables or cereals, coffee beans or hard tropical fruits like avocado and coconut, nothing can withstand its razor sharp blades moving at 24000 rotations per minute.

You can use a nutribullet to process anything which is why this beautiful machine is best suited for making smoothies of different kinds. Since you won't have any problem with blending your ingredients in just a few seconds, you can use it to try all kinds of smoothie recipes with unique ingredients. The best thing about a nutribullet is that it crushes the cell walls of food particles and allows your body to absorb and digest a load of beneficial nutrients.

So what are you waiting for? Buy yourself a nutribullet and try out the recipes in this book. I guarantee that you'll be amazed by the results of your experimentation.

4. Smoothie Recipes for a Healthy Heart

Health problems are increasing every year, thanks to fast food and unhealthy lifestyle. But there is still an easiest and tastiest way to overcome this problem and to keep your heart healthy, happy and loving. It's not hard like exercise and it is also not yucky like medicines. Here are some yummy smoothie recipes that'll keep your heart healthy. You just have to grab some fruits and vegetables and blend them.

Avocado and Blueberry Smoothie

This smoothie recipe should be your number one choice because it is packed with disease fighting phytochemicals and anti-oxidants from blueberries and it also provides you with mono unsaturated fatty acids which are the 'good' fats. Avocados are rich in these 'good' fats and they are famous for lowering LDL which is the 'bad' cholesterol and it increases the level of HDL which is the 'good' cholesterol. Aside from this talk of good and bad cholesterol, avocados are a good source of vitamin B-6 and folic acid which too provide good heart support. **Ingredients**

- Avocado – 1//4

- Blueberries – 1 cup

- Lime juice (half lemon)

- Coconut water – 1 cup

- Honey – 1 Tbsp

Blend until it is nice and smooth.

Acai Berry and Chia Seed Smoothie

Acai seeds can be easily purchased in the form of frozen packets from any drug store. They too are rich in anti-oxidants just like a heart-friendly food. They are also helpful in preventing atherosclerosis. Chia seeds are also good for heart's health because they help in reducing blood pressure. Omega-3 fatty acids in chia seeds are useful for keeping your heart healthy.

Ingredients

- Frozen Acai berries – 3.5 ounces

- Chia seeds – 2 Tbs.

- Unsweetened almond milk – 2 cups

- Liquid stevia – to taste

First, blend milk and berries at low speed to break down the berries. Then blend the mixture at high speed until it is smooth. After that, add chia seeds and stevia. Adjust the sweetness according to your taste.

Berry, Banana and Spinach Smoothie

Berries are very nutritious and they have anti-oxidants which as we all know are essential for a healthy heart. Banana is a great source of potassium which keeps blood pressure in control and spinach has something called Co-Q10 which is useful in the prevention and treatment of cardiovascular disease. Hemp is a good ingredient to improve cardiovascular health.

Ingredients

- Hemp protein powder – 4 Tbs.

- Almond milk – 1 cup

- Berries – half cup

- 1 banana

- 1 handful spinach

Blend properly and enjoy.

Green Lemonade

This green lemonade is a must try because it offers a great many benefits to your heart. Apples contain compounds that delay the breakdown of LDL i.e. bad cholesterol. Lemons help in boosting the immune system and reducing weight. Since obesity is one of the major causes of heart diseases, lemons are great for this purpose. Greens such as spinach, mint, kale, collard, coriander, chard etc. are also said to be really beneficial for heart, especially spinach because it is rich in potassium, iron, fiber, lutein and folate.

Ingredients

- 2 green apples

- 1 handful of greens

- A half peeled lemon

Blend all ingredients and drink immediately.

Heart-Friendly Smoothie

Potassium and calcium in milk and yoghurt help in reducing weight by making you feel full and satisfied. These elements also help in lowering the blood pressure. Cocoa beans are also good for promoting a healthy heart circulation as they contain flavanol. Last but not least, almonds increase the level of HDL and reduce the level of LDL. Hmmm…This really is a heart-friendly smoothie. An interesting name for a smoothie, isn't it?

Ingredients

- Skim milk – half cup

- Nonfat yoghurt – half cup

- 1 banana

- Raspberries – half cup

- Almond butter – 1 Tbs.

- Sweetened dark cocoa powder – 1 Tbsp

- 3 ice cubes

Combine them in nutribullet and blend them well.

Tropical Fruit Smoothie

Everyone likes fruits and if combined together, they are mouth-watering. Oranges, bananas, berries, papaya and grapes makes a sensational smoothie. Besides taste, fruits are good for your heart's health due to a treasure reserve of healthy elements present in them.

Ingredients

- 1 banana

- 1 cup blueberries

- 1 papaya

- 1 cup red grape juice

- 1 cup orange juice

- 1 cup carrot juice

Place all these amazing ingredients in nutribullet, blend and enjoy!

Pomegranate-Blueberry Smoothie

Pomegranate has such a bright and beautiful color like some precious stone. It is one of the best fruits to keep you healthy and to cure your diseases. It is a very powerful anti-oxidant just like blueberries. It restrains abnormal platelet growth to reduce cardiac and stroke risks and it also reduces cholesterol and blood pressure.

Ingredients

- Pure pomegranate juice – half cup

- Unsweetened, frozen berries – 3/4 cup

- Lemon zest – 1/2 teaspoon

- Fresh lemon juice – 1/2 teaspoon

- Nonfat vanilla yoghurt – 1/4 cup

- 3 to 4 ice cubes

First, add all the ingredients except ice. Blend until they are smooth. Then add the ice cubes and blend until it is crushed and looks yummy. Enjoy this splendid drink.

5. Appetizing Detox Smoothies

You have no need to pinch your nose while drinking these delectable detox smoothies. That's right! These are one of the most delicious yet very healthy detox smoothie recipes. They are packed with anti-oxidants which neutralize free radicals and cleanse your body. So, experience the richness and flavor of all the ingredients while you give your body what it needs. There you go with some super recipes.

Happy Berry Breakfast

Enjoy this wonderful detox smoothie which is packed with a punch of anti-oxidants! Oh! And honey will purify your body from inside out, giving your skin a nice glow.

Ingredients

- Unsweetened, frozen raspberries – 1 cup

- Frozen unsweetened cherries – 1/4 cup

- Freshly grated ginger – 2 tsp

- Unsweetened, chilled almond milk – 3/4 cup

- Honey – 1 Tbsp

- Fresh lemon juice – 2 tsp

- Ground flaxseed – 1 tsp

Combine them all in a blender. Blend and enjoy.

Green Smoothie

Greens are full of iron and elements that wipe out all the toxics from your body. Plus they are rich in fiber which eliminates all the chances of constipation. You will feel really good if you try this recipe.

Ingredients

- Chopped kale leaves – 1/4 cup

- Mango cubes – 1 cup

- 2 chopped medium ribbed celery

- Fresh orange juice – 1 cup

- Fresh chopped mint – 1/4 cup

- Chopped parsley – 1/4 cup

Blend them nice and smooth and have a drink.

Kale Smoothie

Kale and ginger, a great combination! Ginger is good for digestion and kale has all the qualities which are possessed by green vegetables.

Ingredients

- Kale – 1 cup

- Half pear

- 1/4 avocado

- Half lemon

- Half cucumber

- Coconut water – half cup

- Ginger – half inch

- 1 scoop protein powder (pea, pumpkin or hemp)

- Water

Blend them and there you have a healthy drink.

Alkalinity Delight

As you can see from the name, this recipe will neutralize the acidity in the stomach and give you a really soothing feeling.

Ingredients

- Half pear

- 1 cup spinach

- 1/4 avocado

- 1 cup almond milk

- 1/4 cup coconut water

- 1 scoop protein powder

- 1 teaspoon chia seeds Blend them well.

Papaya Smoothie

Papayas are rich in vitamins C and E. These vitamins and coconut kefir together makes a good detox smoothie. Coconut kefir has a healthy dose of probiotics which are good for your stomach.

Ingredients

- Papaya – 1 cup

- Juice from a half lime

- Coconut kefir – 1 cup

- Raw honey – 1 Tbsp

Such an easy recipe! Blend them and sooth your belly with this light smoothie.

Smooth Vitamin C and Fiber

This recipe contains a root vegetable called jicama which is rich in vitamin C.

Ingredients
- Jicama – half cup

- 5 romaine lettuce leaves

- Half cucumber

- 1/4 avocado

- A handful of cilantro

- 1 date
- Hemp protein – 4 scoops

- 1 whole lime Blend well.

Morning Freshness

If you make cucumber the base of your detox smoothie, it's a wise choice. It not only hydrates your body but it is also alkaline in nature. It provides you with some minerals as well.

Ingredients

- 1 cucumber

- 2 stalks of celery

- A fistful of romaine

- A fistful of kale

- 1 green apple

- 1 broccoli stem

- Half peeled lemon

Wash and cut all ingredients. After that, make a nice juice/shake and freshen up yourself.

Cranberry Smoothie

Try this brilliant cranberry smoothie not only to detox your body but also to keep your kidneys strong. It is rich in vitamin C, E, K, manganese and a large number of phytonutrients which keeps you miles and miles away from urinary tract infection, cardiovascular disease, cancer and dental problems. Say hello to this remarkable smoothie!

Ingredients

- Cranberries – half cup

- 1 cucumber

- 1 pear

- 1 apple

- 1 celery stalk

- A handful of spinach

Juice them all and take advantage of this very healthy smoothie.

6. Smoothie Recipes for Improved Energy

If you need to boost your energy, smoothies are a great and instant way of doing that. Don't go for coffee, tea or an artificial energy drink to give you a kick start. Instead go for the healthier options like a nourishing glass of smoothie. In the presence of such energy boosting smoothies you need not worry about your weakening immune system. They are rich in carbohydrates, proteins, calcium, vitamins, minerals and a lot more to increase the energy reserves of your body.

Fresh Morning Smoothie

Vitamin C, anti-oxidants, carbohydrates and great flavor are what make this an ideal morning smoothie.

Ingredients

- Fresh tangerine juice of 3 tangerines

- A handful of frozen strawberries

- Fresh juice of a red grapefruit

Mix the strawberries with the juice of tangerines and grapefruit and blend the mixture. This delicious and very easy recipe will bring smile on your face. Got to try it!

Blueberry-Mango Smoothie

Blueberry is a wonderful source of anti-oxidants and mango is the king. Mangoes are a good source of Caretenoids and vitamin C which help in boosting the immune system. Apart from these advantages, this smoothie contains bananas which are known to be an instant source of energy.

Ingredients

- 1 pint of blueberries

- 1 mango

- 1 banana

- 1 cup of almond milk

- 1 tsp of maple syrup

Chop the mangoes and then blend all the ingredients in a blender. Your energizing drink is ready. Add some ice if you like.

Berry Berry

Berries are popular in smoothies not just because they look good and they taste good but because they have so much more to offer in terms of improving your health. They have disease fighting phytochemicals, specifically blueberries. Berries are also a rich source of anti-oxidants, as mentioned time and again. Honey is also an important energy boosting ingredient, sweet but way better than the processed sugar.

Ingredients

- Blueberries – half cup

- Blackberries – half cup

- Cherries – half cup

- 1 banana

- Honey – 1 tsp

- Almond milk – 1 cup

- Flaxseed oil – 1 Tbsp

- Dash of cinnamon

Blend them until you see the smooth and creamy texture.

Strawberry Smoothie

Strawberries boost immunity! How? They are an excellent source of vitamin C which is a well-known immunity booster and also a great anti-oxidant. You can get your daily requirement of Vitamin C from this smoothie.

Ingredients

- Strawberries – 1 cup

- 1 sliced frozen banana

- Coconut milk – 1 cup

- Honey – 1 tsp

Puree them in your blender and take your much needed vitamin C.

Peach Smoothie

Peaches combat diseases including cancer and they also lower the risk of heart diseases. They give you an amazing boost of energy and nourish your skin as well.

Ingredients
- 1 peach

- Strawberries / raspberries – half cup

- Low fat peach yogurt – half cup

- Milk – 1/4 cup

Peel and chop the peach and pop all the ingredients in your blender. Now what? Grab a glass and drink.

Melon Smoothie

Dehydrated after exercise or some tough physical work? This melon smoothie will hydrate you as water melon contains 92% water and make you feel fresh again.

- Watermelon cubes – 1 cup

- Honeydew melon cubes – half cup

- Cantaloupe cubes – 1 cup

- Frozen strawberries – 1 cup

Blend them until it is smooth and freshen up with this rich drink.

Fruit Luxury

Fruits provide you with all the energy if you cut on your diet to reduce weight. You won't feel weak and you will not gain weight if you try this smoothie recipe. This smoothie is made of pineapples, oranges, berries and bananas. Combine all the benefits and you get a wonderful source of energy.

Ingredients

- 5 slices of pineapple

- 1 banana

- 2 oranges

- A handful of berries

- 1/4 cup of water

- Some ice

Peel and section the oranges. Juice the oranges and pineapple and add water. Then add all the ingredients. Start on low speed to crush the ice and then speed up to make a smooth drink. You will feel like you are on a beach enjoying a nice and refreshing drink.

Kiwi Smoothie

Kiwi is also one of the keys to boost your immune system because it contains twice the amount of vitamin C than oranges. It is also a good source of potassium which will keep your heart healthy and strong. This recipe has two more ingredients which will give strength to your immune system, mangoes and the algae called Spirulina. So, this recipe will give you 3 times more energy than eating a single fruit.

Ingredients

- 2 kiwis

- 1 mango

- 2 tsp Spirulina powder

- 100 ml of coconut milk

- 2 tsp honey

- 75 ml of low fat yoghurt

Peel and chop mango and kiwis. Add into the blender along with the coconut milk. Blend until the fruit is mixed. Then add the rest of the ingredients and keep the machine on until it is smooth. Add some ice and drink to your heart's delight.

7. Smoothie Recipes for Beautiful Skin

Are you tired of using different kinds of skin freshness creams and lotions that still haven't produced your desired results? If yes, then throw those useless things out the window right away and go for something that really works. I'm talking about yummy smoothies made of fresh fruits and vegetables. The amount of skin freshening nutrients in these recipes is enormous.

The Green Beauty Smoothie:

Lettuce, parsley and apples with bananas and kale is a conventional yet exceedingly enticing recipe that will make you feel lighter. The cleansing agents in these ingredients will take good care of your skin.

Ingredients:

- 4 lettuce leaves

- 1 baby kale

- 4 sprays of parsley

- A small lemon

- A Fuji apple

- A banana

- 2 TB of flax seeds mixed with chia seeds

- Half a glass of water

- 4 ice cubes

- 1/16 table spoon of stevia

Add kale, romaine, apple, parsley, lemon, cucumber, ginger, and water to your blender. After that close the lid and switch on your blender. Turn up the variable knob to 10. The contents would be broken down in about 15-20 seconds. Then add the remaining ingredients to the blender. Blend the mixture for 1 minute. Your Green Beauty Smoothie will be ready for you to enjoy it.

Healthy Skin Berry Smoothie:

A cool looking smoothie that contains all the "winning ingredients"! The freshness of berries coupled with the taste of yogurt and flaxseeds will surely have you captivated. And, there is no denying to the fact berries are like "ninjas" against oxidants and other unpleasant substances that are harmful for your skin.

Ingredients:

- ½ bowl of blueberries

- ¼ bowl of raspberries

- ¼ bowl of strawberries

- ¼ bowl of kale

- 1 fat free pack of yogurt

- 1 TSP honey

- 2 TSP flax seeds

- ½ cup water

Add these ingredients in your blender. Blend for about 2 minutes and then enjoy the smooth creamy drink.

Coconut Water and Strawberry Smoothie:

Chilly coconut water, fresh strawberries and oranges… can't get better than that on a hot sunny day! The coconut water will keep your skin fresh by supporting the fatty acids beneath it and the strawberries will fulfill your vitamin C deficiency.

Ingredients:

- A cup of chilled coconut water

- A small bowl of fresh strawberries

- 1 cup of organic carrots

- A cup of fresh mango pieces

- A peeled naval orange

Add these things in your blender along with some ice to make a real smooth and chilly drink.

Almond Banana Delight:

An unbelievably tasty and appetizing smoothie! It's a perfect combination of almonds and bananas that will prove be a perfect start for a busy summer day.

Ingredients:

- A frozen banana in small pieces'

- 1 TSP of peanut butter

- 2 TSP of flax seeds

- ½ cup of milk

- A drizzle of maple syrup

- A drop of almond or vanilla extract

Berry Beauty Smoothie:

A beautiful and delectable combination of strawberries and blueberries that will have you hooked right away. These along with some other novel ingredients are the perfect skin cleansing tools.

Ingredients:

- ¼ cup of frozen strawberries and same quantity of blueberries

- One peeled orange

- A banana

- ½ cup of plain yogurt

- Silken tofu, ½ cup

- 2 TSP chia seeds and 1 TSP agave nectar

Just blend until it gets smooth and enjoy it while relaxing, reading a novel or watching TV.

Superb Complexion Smoothie:

The usage of simple ingredients like kale and spinach gives this smoothie a great flavor and makes it extremely healthy. Kale is a medically proven vegetable that helps in making your complexion fair. Besides kale, this smoothie is packed with a load of nutritious and scrumptious elements.

Ingredients:

- A cup of both spinach and kale leaves

- A cup of green grapes

- A pear with its seeds, core and stem removed

- 1 orange and 1 banana, both peeled

- 1 TSP chia seeds

- ½ cup of water

- 1 glass ice

Put all the ingredients in your blender and blend at slow speed for about 20 seconds. Then move to medium and high speed within the next 60 seconds. In less than 2 minutes, you'll have yourself a wonderful green smoothie.

Avocado Smoothie:

Composed of avocado and other fruits, this smoothie is loaded with vitamins E, C and K that are needed for maintaining healthy and fresh skin. And if you are suffering from skin inflammation, this smoothie is the right thing for you.

Ingredients:

- One ripe peach

- Chopped Avocado, 2 tablespoon

- 4-5 frozen strawberries

- About ½ cup of fat-free yogurt

- 3 tsp pomegranate juice
- Grape-seed oil and vanilla extract, 1 tsp each

Puree all ingredients in your blender until smooth. Best have it after a workout and replenish your lost minerals.

8. Smoothie Recipes for Weight Loss

Achieving that perfect figure seems really hard…Think…think…what to do to reduce the undesired fat from your body? The answer is not that complicated. That's right! Don't worry about complex menus to reduce weight which don't really give the choice of good taste. Here is a variety of smoothies which are easy to make and are a best source to incorporate fresh fruits and vegetables. These smoothie recipes also provide you with the much needed mono unsaturated fatty acids which aim to reduce belly fat. They are creamy, rich and perfect for breakfast, lunch or as a snack.

Mango Surprise

Who says that you need to completely cut out the sweet flavor in order to reduce weight? This smoothie will satisfy your hunger for something sweet and at the same time reduce weight. Mangoes have high fiber and water content. That's why they not only help prevent constipation but fiber makes you feel full and satisfied for a long time. This is the key to reduce weight: take a lot of fiber.

Ingredients

- Mango cubes – 1/4 cup

- Mango juice – 1/2 cup

- Avocado – 1/4 cup

- Fresh lime juice – 1 Tbsp

- 6 ice cubes

Process them in a blender and garnish with any fruit if you like.

Purple Smoothie

Blueberries are low on sugar content and rich in fiber. They are more than perfect to shed some extra pounds. This recipe's star is blueberry.

Ingredients

- Unsweetened, frozen blueberries – 1 cup

- Skim milk – 1 cup

- Cold-pressed, organic flax seed oil – 1 Tbsp

Blend blueberries and skim milk for 1 minute. Pour in the glass and mix the oil.

Banana Boom

This amazing fruit is packed with all those superb nutrients to keep you smart and healthy. If combined with calcium rich food like yogurt and milk, you wouldn't need anything else.

Ingredients

- 1 banana

- Plain fat-free yogurt – half cup

- Fat-free milk – half cup

- Unsalted peanut butter – 2 Tbsp

- Honey- 1 Tbsp

- 4 ice cubes

Combine all ingredients in a blender and process until it becomes a fine shake.

Blueberry and Vanilla Yogurt Smoothie

This smoothie is perfect for you to lose weight because it offers fiber, richness of yogurt and that amazing vanilla flavor. You wouldn't miss your ice cream if you try this.

Ingredients

- 1 cup frozen blueberries

- 6 ounce vanilla yogurt

- 1 cup skim milk

- 1 tablespoon flaxseed oil

Shake all the ingredients in a blender except flaxseed oil. When shaken properly, pour in a glass and mix the flaxseed oil.

Raspberry and Chocolate Smoothie

Huh! Chocolate! Well, don't be surprised. This isn't any sweet chocolate which will make you look like a bear. This smoothie recipe includes chocolate chips in a small quantity which will provide you with mono unsaturated fatty acids i.e. the healthy fats. They will make your smoothie satisfying and help your body absorb vitamins.

Ingredients

- Fresh Raspberries – 1 cup

- Chocolate chips – 1/4 cup

- Skim milk – half cup

- Vanilla yogurt – 6 oz

- Frozen raspberries – 1 cup

Blend for 1 minute and relish this smoothie any time.

Peachy Shake

Refreshing and light, is what can be said about this smoothie. The main fruit in this recipe is perfect for achieving that ideal body weight and also give a fresh tone to your skin.

Ingredients

- Frozen, unsweetened peaches – 1 cup

- Skim milk – 1 cup

- Cold-pressed organic flaxseed oil – 2 Tbsp

Always add flaxseed oil in the glass after shaking the ingredients. Such an easy way to become slim and smart!

Citrus Smoothie

Citrus fruits such as orange and lemon are highly recommended when you are struggling to lose that stubborn body fat which makes you look older than your age.

Ingredients

- 1 orange

- Lemon Yogurt – 6 oz

- Skim milk – 1 cup

- Flaxseed oil – 1 Tbsp

- Some ice

Peel and section the orange and pop everything in the blender except flaxseed oil. Add the oil after processing the ingredients. This smoothie will make you feel good.

9. Anti-Aging Smoothies

There are so many stories about the fountain of youth, how people try to get there, and all that aura of romance surrounding these stories. While listening to and reading these stories some of you must have thought about that pure beauty and youth which catches the eye at once. Here is the news for you; you can make your own fountain of youth. That's right! There are some things which will slow down your aging process and make you look a lot younger. Anti-aging smoothies are that fountain of youth that you can make with some ingredients and the push of a button. Magic! Isn't it? These smoothies contain those ingredients which will improve your overall health and give your skin a nice glow. Here are some amazing recipes for you.

Healthy Beauty

This smoothie delivers a lot of vitamins, minerals and immune boosting nutrients. Chia seeds, tofu and yogurt provide you with calcium, proteins and iron to reduce inflammation and protect and maintain cell membranes. A+ Grade for the fruits because they help in building skin-firming collagen, rebuilds skin cells and work against oxidative damage. Drink for health and beauty.

Ingredients

- Blueberries – half cup

- Strawberries – 1/4 cup

- 1 banana

- 1 orange

- Tofu – half cup

- Fat-free plain yogurt – half cup

- Agave nectar – 1 tsp

- Chia seeds – 2 Tbsp

Prep all the fruits and whip all ingredients until smooth. Drink and think about regaining the splendor of youth.

Kale and Spinach Smoothie

The secret behind gorgeous skin – kale! It's full of carotenoids which gives your skin a healthy touch and makes it glow. Not only that, it also protects your skin from wrinkles. Drinking this smoothie is a perfect way to look attractive.

Ingredients

- Kale – 1 cup

- Spinach – 1cup

- Green seedless grapes – 1cup

- 1 pear

- 1 banana

- 1 orange

- Chia seeds – 1 tsp

- Water – half cup

- Ice – 2 cups

Chop kale, spinach and pear. Peel banana and orange and remove the seeds of orange. Place all the ingredients in nutribullet and blend on low speed for 15 seconds. Then process on medium speed and then on high speed until everything is nice and smooth.

Coconut Smoothie

Beauty tips are not all about applying sun block, different cosmetics and even natural ingredients over your skin. There is no denying that these things help but you need something more. Something in the diet perhaps can help you gain awesome loveliness and heath at the same time. Including smoothies in your diet is the easiest way to look pretty. Coconut smoothie is one of the crucial drinks because coconut contains healthy fats. The presence of lauric acid in coconut oil gives it antimicrobial properties. Vitamin E in coconut is good for skin repair and growth. Last but not least, the saturated fat in coconut oil even protects the skin from UV damage. Include this amazing fruit in your smoothies and gain youth like beauty.

Ingredients

- 1 Sustain packet

- Shredded unsweetened coconut – 1 Tbsp

- Coconut oil – 1 Tbsp

- Unsweetened almond milk – 4 oz

- Water – 4 oz

- Half banana

- 4 ice cubes

Blend all ingredients and enjoy the taste of youth.

Avocado and Strawberry Smoothie

Here are the avocados! You must be thinking: "Yeah, what do they do?" and "What's the excitement for?" Let me tell you, they are loaded with vitamins C, E, and K which are very important for healthy skin. They also help in reducing dryness and irritation. Moreover, they contain glutathione which blocks intestinal absorption of certain fats that cause damage to the skin. Now what do you think?

Ingredients

- Chopped Hass avocado – 2 Tbsp

- 1 peach

- Unsweetened frozen strawberries – 1/3 cup

- Pure pomegranate juice – 3 Tbsp

- Fat-free plain yoghurt – 3/4 cup

- Vanilla extract – 1 tsp

- Grapeseed oil – 1 tsp

Puree all ingredients well in a blender. It must be yummy.

Berry Blast

It you want to make your skin perfect from inside out, try some berries. Berries are packed with anti-oxidants which neutralize the free radicals that damage our skin cells. Hydrating water and vitamin C in the berries are essential for a healthy complexion. Do you want to know more? They also help the body manufacture collagen which gives your skin a flawless beauty.

Ingredients

- Raspberries – 1/4 cup

- Blueberries – 1/4 cup

- Strawberries – 1/4 cup

- Kale – 1/4 cup

- Water – 1 cup

Just crush these ingredients in your blender and get numerous benefits.

Tropical Vacation

Composed of a lot of wonderful fruits, this smoothie will make you fee. that you are on vacation in the Caribbean. Mango and pineapple in this smoothie will slow down the aging process because of vitamin C, beta carotene and omega 3.

Ingredients

- 2 mangoes

- Half pineapple

- 2 kiwis

- Orange juice – 1 cup

- 3 ice cubes

Whirl them in your blender, take a sip and imagine the view of the beach…

Keep Me Active Smoothie

This smoothie will remove dark circles, keep you active and energetic. Must try!

- Blueberries – 1 cup

- Raspberries – 2 cups

- Flaxseed powder – 2 Tbsp

- Goji berry powder – 1 Tbsp

- Kefir – 1 cup

Hopefully, you'll appreciate the energetic punch of this smoothie.

Fountain of Youth

This anti-aging smoothie will make you smart and healthy. Bananas in this smoothie will aid with digestion and green tea powder will keep you active, combat inflammation and reduce the risk of diseases because it contains polyphenols and caffeine. The coconut water and strawberries will illuminate your skin. How cool!

Ingredients

- Strawberries – 3 cups

- Green tea powder – 1 Tbsp

- 1 banana

- Chia seed powder – 2 Tbsp

- Coconut powder – 1 cup

Combine all these beneficial ingredients and process in your blender. Your smoothie is ready.

10. Superfood Smoothies

We hear the term "superfoods" a lot these days but we don't really know what these are? Let me tell you that these foods are rich in nutrients that our bodies need but don't receive. The most common superfoods are chia seeds, flax seeds, coconut oil, spirulina, cacao nibs, avocado, hemp protein, camu powder and acai. A lot of us usually use these foods in meals and snacks but they can be used in smoothies as well. In fact, a smoothie composed of superfoods will boost up your stamina and make you really energetic.

Choco-Berry Almond Smoothie

It has chocolate, almond milk, blueberries and a bunch of other exciting ingredients which make it a worthy meal replacement.

Ingredients

- A cup of almond milk

- Frozen blueberries, raspberries and soaked almonds, ¼ cup each

- 1 tablespoon butter

- 1 TSP cacao powder

- Cinnamon and vanilla extract, ¼ tablespoon

- 1 TSP of honey

The Dream Smoothie

This recipe has all the dreamy ingredients. Avocado, blueberries, almonds, you name it! Whether you are exhausted after a harsh workout or drained after a long day at work, this smoothie will rock you up.

Ingredients:

- A cup of almond milk

- ½ cup fat-free yogurt

- ½ piece of avocado
- ½ cup of blueberries, frozen preferably

- 2-3 Brazil nuts

- 1 TSP cacao powder

- 1 TSP cacao nibs

- 1 TSP maca

- 1 TSP lucuma

- 1/4 TSP cinnamon

- 2-3 drops of vanilla extract

- A serving of protein powder of your choice

Blend all ingredients in your nutribullet until smooth.

Spirulina with Chocolate and Blueberry Smoothie:

A real hardcore smoothie with a perfect combination of blueberries and spirulina! Now you can have your vitamins and minerals all in one glass of this smoothie.

Ingredients:

- A cup of milk

- One-third of an avocado

- Half a cup of frozen blueberries

- 1 TSP of both tahini and cacao powder

- ½ TSP cacao nibs

- ½ TSP spirulina

- ½ TSP vanilla extract

- ½ TSP honey

Just blend all the ingredients until smooth and knock yourself out!

Cacao Acai Smoothie

If you want to save yourself from cancer, premature aging other kinds of nasty diseases, then grab your blender and follow this recipe right away. The acai and cacao nibs in this smoothie recipe are full of antioxidants that kill free radicals and other bad boys that may cause harm to your body.

Ingredients

- Coconut water, 1 cup

- 1/3 avocado

- 1/2 cup of yogurt

- 1/2 cup of strawberries

- 1 TSP butter

- 1 TSP cacao powder

- 1 TSP blended goji berries

- Chia seeds, bee pollen and acai powder, 1 teaspoon each

- 1/4 teaspoon of cinnamon

- A pinch of sea salt

- 1/2 tablespoon of honey

Aloe Vera Citrus Smoothie

Aloe Vera is the champion of herbs because of its amazing medicinal characteristics. It helps in detoxification, improving immunity, digestion, countering inflammations and carcinogenic substances, skin freshness and above all it's a heart friendly herb. With so much to offer, it would be unwise not to use this splendid herb in a smoothie.

Ingredients

- 1 cup water

- 1/3 avocado

- A medium sized aloe vera leaf

- A small sized lemon, peeled

- 1 TSP coconut oil

- A dash of salt

- One tablespoon honey

- 4-5 ice cubes

Add all the ingredients in your nutribullet and blend for about 45 seconds. Pour it in a glass and garnish it with a peeled kiwi and half tablespoon of flax seeds.

Banana Delight Smoothie

Who doesn't like a creamy banana smoothie on a hot summer eve? I wouldn't have second thoughts about not having it, would you? The chilly banana, fresh strawberries and mango chunks will make it difficult for you to stop.

Ingredients

- About 200g of almond milk

- 1 frozen banana

- A cup of spinach

- Frozen mango chunks and strawberries, 1/2 cup each

- 2 TSP Greek yogurt

- 1 TSP coconut oil

- 1 TSP chia gel

- 1 TSP bee pollen

Blend until smooth and let it cool you off!

The Energizer

The name speaks for itself! Whenever you need something to fill you up with immense energy, go for "The Energizer." Being composed of tropical fruits, berries and green vegetables, this recipe is a reservoir of vitamins, proteins and carbohydrates.

Ingredients

- A cup of coconut water

- Half avocado

- Half cup of tropical fruits like pineapple, mango and papaya

- 1/2 bowl of spinach

- Kale, 1/2 cup

- ½ cup Greek yogurt

- Goji berries and cranberries, 2 tablespoon each

- Coconut oil, coconut flakes, maca, 1 teaspoon each

- 1 teaspoon of wheatgrass powder

- 1 tablespoon honey

Blend all the ingredients for about 45 seconds. Pour in a glass and drink up!

11. THANK YOU FOR READING!

Thank You so much for reading this book. If this title gave you a ton of value, It would be amazing for you to leave a REVIEW !

THANK YOU FOR DOWNLOADING! IF YOU ENJOYED THIS BOOK AND WOULD LIKE TO READ MORE TITLES FROM MY COLLECTION CLICK THIS LINK